STOMACH CANCER AWARENESS BOOKLET

EMPOWERING SUPPORT & INFORMATION FOR YOU & LOVED ONES. WE CAN BEAT CANCER TOGETHER!
JOIN THE MOVEMENT

WRITTEN BY DELATRIA SAM

AF715355

Stomach Cancer Awareness Booklet © 2025 by Delatria Sam
All rights reserved.
No part of this publication may be reproduced, distributed, or transmitted in any form or by any means, including photocopying, recording, or other electronic or mechanical methods, without the prior written permission of the publisher or author, except as permitted by U.S. copyright law.
ISBN: 979-8-3495-6750-6

Dear Friend,

November is recognized as Stomach Cancer Awareness Month, a time dedicated to raising awareness, sharing knowledge, extending empathy and compassion to those affected by stomach cancer. Whether you are someone navigating a diagnosis, a caregiver, a family member, or a friend, please know this: you are not alone.

This booklet was intended and created as both an informative resource and a gentle companion. Inside, you'll find:

- Clear information about stomach cancer, its symptoms, treatment options, and more
- Journaling prompts to encourage reflection and emotional release
- Coloring pages and creative activities designed to reduce stress and provide comfort
-FAQs: Frequently Asked Questions about Stomach Cancer
-Quotes: Inspirational quotes about hope and resilience
-Games and Puzzles: Word search, word scramble, & brain teasers to learn about cancer
- Words of encouragement and support to remind you of your strength and tenacity
-Nutrition and Wellness information, food & beverage diary tracker
-Patient Empowerment Tip
-Research Updates
-Diagram of the digestive system to help explain how stomach cancer develops
-Survivor and caregiver tips
-Cancer Wish List: A heartfelt section where you can write wishes, hopes, or prayers
-Self-care compass
-Dialogue: A conversation between a patient, the healthcare provider, and caregivers
-Love Letters: Heartfelt letters from a survivor to themselves, loved ones, and caregivers
-Medical Glossary: Definitions of key medical terms related to stomach cancer
-Thank you letter & In loving memory page

I hope that these pages provide not only information but also comfort, rest, and hope. Life with or around stomach cancer can often feel overwhelming. My wish is that this booklet provides you with the knowledge, comfort, rest, and hope you need during this challenging time.

To the Caregivers...
Your love, dedication, and tireless efforts do not go unnoticed. You are the unsung heroes, providing comfort, support, and care to those navigating the challenges of stomach cancer.

To my loved ones who lost their lives to stomach cancer...
Your memory lives on in my heart, and I hope that this booklet will bring comfort, strength, and hope to those who are walking a similar path. May your legacy inspire us to fight for a future where stomach cancer is better understood, treated, and ultimately defeated.

With love and support,
Delatria Sam
Author of "5 Essential Insights into Stomach Cancer: Supporting Yourself and Loved Ones"

Stomach Cancer

As someone working in the health and medicine sector, it's essential to understand what stomach cancer is and its implications. Stomach cancer, also known as gastric cancer, is a serious disease that affects thousands of individuals worldwide. It's crucial to raise awareness about this often-overlooked disease to promote early detection, support patients and families, advocate for research, and seek better treatment options.

Stomach cancer begins when cells in the lining of the stomach grow out of control, forming a tumor. The most common type is adenocarcinoma, which originates in the mucus-producing cells of the stomach lining.

Several factors increase the risk of developing stomach cancer:
- *Helicobacter pylori infection: A bacterial infection that causes ulcers and chronic inflammation*
- *Diet: Consuming salty, smoked, or pickled foods and a low intake of fruits and vegetables*
- *Smoking and tobacco use: Significantly increases the risk of stomach cancer*
- *Family history: Having a close relative with stomach cancer increases the risk*
- *Age: Stomach cancer is more common in people over 60*
- *Previous stomach surgery or polyps: Increases the risk of developing stomach cancer*
- *Race & Ethnicity: Certain racial and ethnic groups may be more susceptible to stomach cancer*

Signs of stomach cancer can be subtle, but common symptoms include:
- *Persistent indigestion or heartburn*
- *Loss of appetite*
- *Nausea and vomiting*
- *Bloating after meals*
- *Stomach pain or discomfort*
- *Blood in stool or black stools*
- *Unexplained weight loss*
- *Fatigue or weakness*
- *Losing interest in activities you once loved*
- *Unsteady gait*
- *Loss of control of bowel movements*
- *Unable to lie down comfortably, having to sleep sitting up*

Your safe space

Think about a place where you felt completely safe and at peace during your journey with stomach cancer. Describe this place in as much detail as you can. What did it look like, sound, and smell like? How did you feel when you were there? Write down any memories or feelings that come to mind when you think about this safe space. How can you bring elements of this space into your current life and help you cope with challenges?

You can express your thoughts and feelings through writing, drawing, painting, or any other form of creative expression that feels meaningful to you.

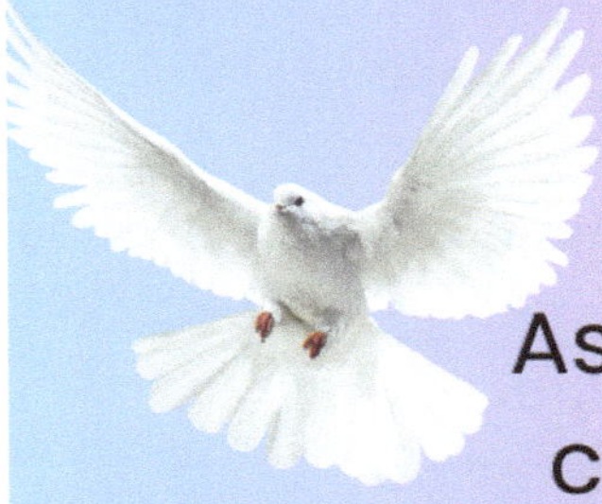

Peace in the Journey

As we journey through the triumphs and challenges of stomach cancer, finding tranquility and peace can be a powerful way to cope with stress and the unknown. By taking moments to breathe, relax, reflect, and find peace, we can cultivate a sense of calmness and resilience that can help us navigate even the most difficult times.

Coloring Activity

To help you find peace and relaxation, we've included a coloring page featuring the word "Peace" and the letter P surrounded by flowers and leaves. Take a moment to color, breathe, and find calm in the present moment.

May this activity bring you a sense of peace and comfort as you navigate your journey.

Peace

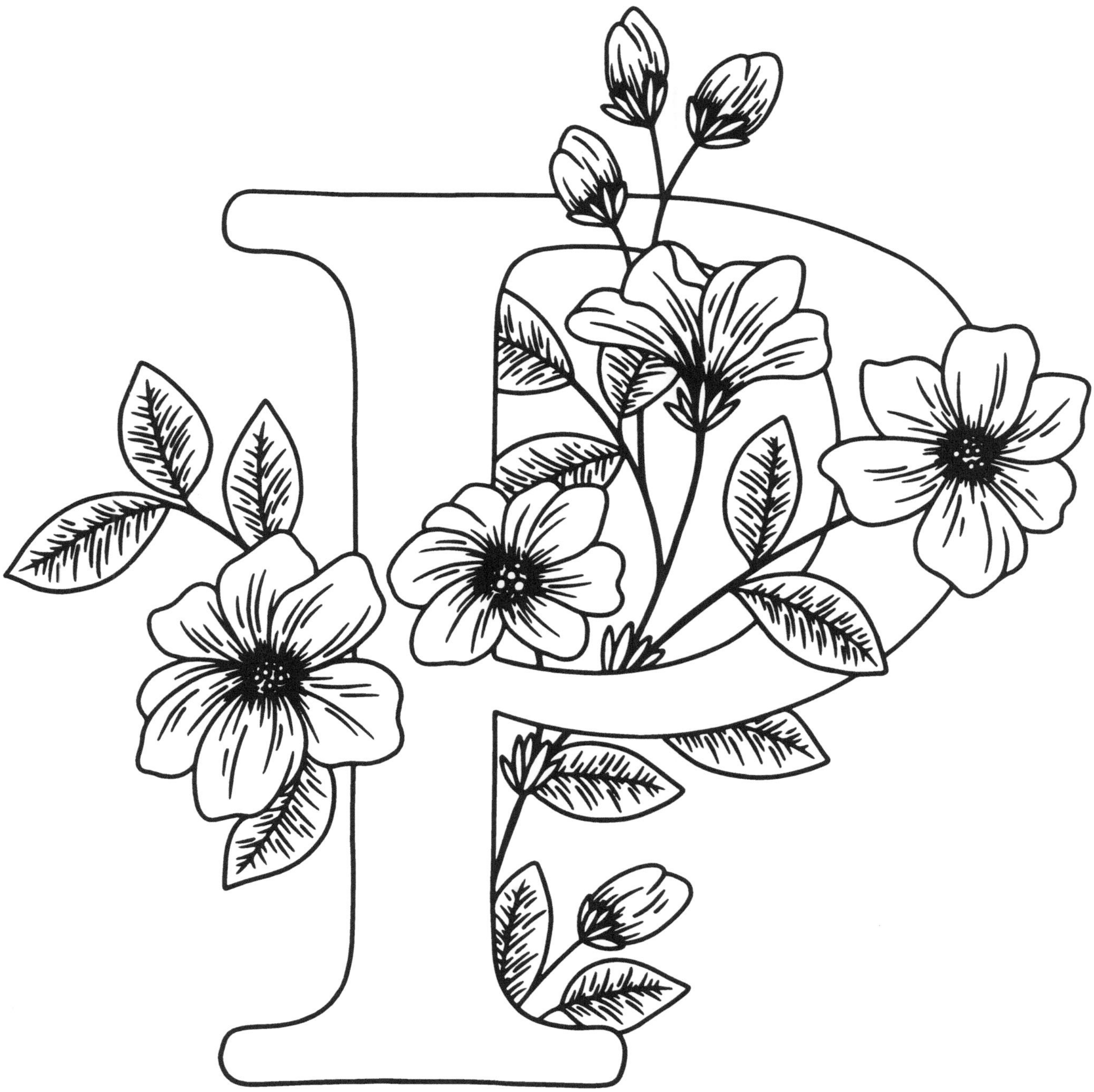

Q&A Time

QUESTION

How can I find strength during cancer treatment?

ANSWER

Draw strength from your support system, self-care practices, and the resilience you've built. Focus on taking things one day at a time and celebrating small victories along the way.

"Healing is a matter of time, but it is sometimes also a matter of opportunity."
~Hippocrates

Stomach Cancer Word Search

R	D	I	A	G	N	O	S	I	S	D
E	E	A	E	E	T	M	U	G	H	O
C	T	M	M	G	H	O	R	A	C	S
N	N	O	T	A	G	T	V	S	R	S
A	E	T	R	R	I	G	I	T	A	E
C	M	P	O	U	F	N	V	R	E	N
C	T	M	P	O	E	I	O	I	S	E
A	A	Y	P	C	V	L	R	C	E	R
R	E	S	U	J	O	A	S	P	R	A
E	R	N	S	A	L	E	O	N	G	W
S	T	O	M	A	C	H	U	X	S	A

Stomach	Treatment	Survivor	Fight
Cancer	Diagnosis	Symptom	Healing
Awareness	Hope	Gastric	Courage
Support	Research	Care	Love

Stomach Cancer

Prevention and Early Detection
While there's no sure way to prevent stomach cancer, lifestyle and dietary choices can help reduce the risk:
- Eat a balanced diet: Focus on fruits, vegetables, and whole grains
- Avoid smoking and tobacco: Reduce your risk of stomach cancer and other health problems
- Manage stress: Chronic stress can negatively impact your health
- Get regular check-ups: Early detection is key to effective treatment. Even if you think you're okay and may have a case of the common cold, it's best to see a doctor early on, rather than waiting too long or until symptoms worsen.

Treatment Options
Treatment depends on the stage, location, and overall health of the cancer, as well as the patient's individual circumstances and medical needs.
-Surgery: To remove the tumor or part of the stomach
-Chemotherapy: To kill cancer cells
-Radiation therapy: To target cancer cells
-Targeted therapy: To target specific cancer cells

Support and Resources
If you or a loved one is affected by stomach cancer, there are resources available to provide support and guidance:
- Cancer Society: Offers information and support for cancer patients and caregivers
- Cancer Institute: Provides information and resources for cancer patients and caregivers
- Local support groups: Provide a community and connection for those affected by stomach cancer
- Speaking with loved ones who may have had a similar experience: Can help cope with the emotional aspects of cancer
- Painting: Can be a great source of therapy and stress relief
- Writing or journaling: Can be a great source of inspiration and emotional release
- Listening to soothing and relaxing music: Can help reduce stress and promote well-being

Strength in the Storm

Write about a time you or a loved one showed strength, courage, or resilience. Reflect on the situation and how strength was shown, emotions experienced, lessons learned, and how this memory reminds you of your ability to endure. Share your story to inspire others!

Finding Strength in the Journey

When life throws us unexpected curveballs, it's easy to feel overwhelmed and want to give up. A stomach cancer diagnosis can be especially daunting, leaving you feeling lost and unsure of what lies ahead. But in the midst of uncertainty, it's the inner strength that can carry you through the darkest moments. It's the resilience that helps you face each new day with courage and hope. You are not alone in this journey. Remember, strength isn't about being unbreakable; it's about finding the courage to keep going, even when the road ahead seems impossible.

Coloring Activity

To help you find strength in the journey, we've included a coloring page featuring the word "Strength" and the letter S surrounded by flowers and leaves. Take a moment to color, breathe, and find comfort in the present moment.

You are stronger than you think, and there is hope to hold onto.

Strength

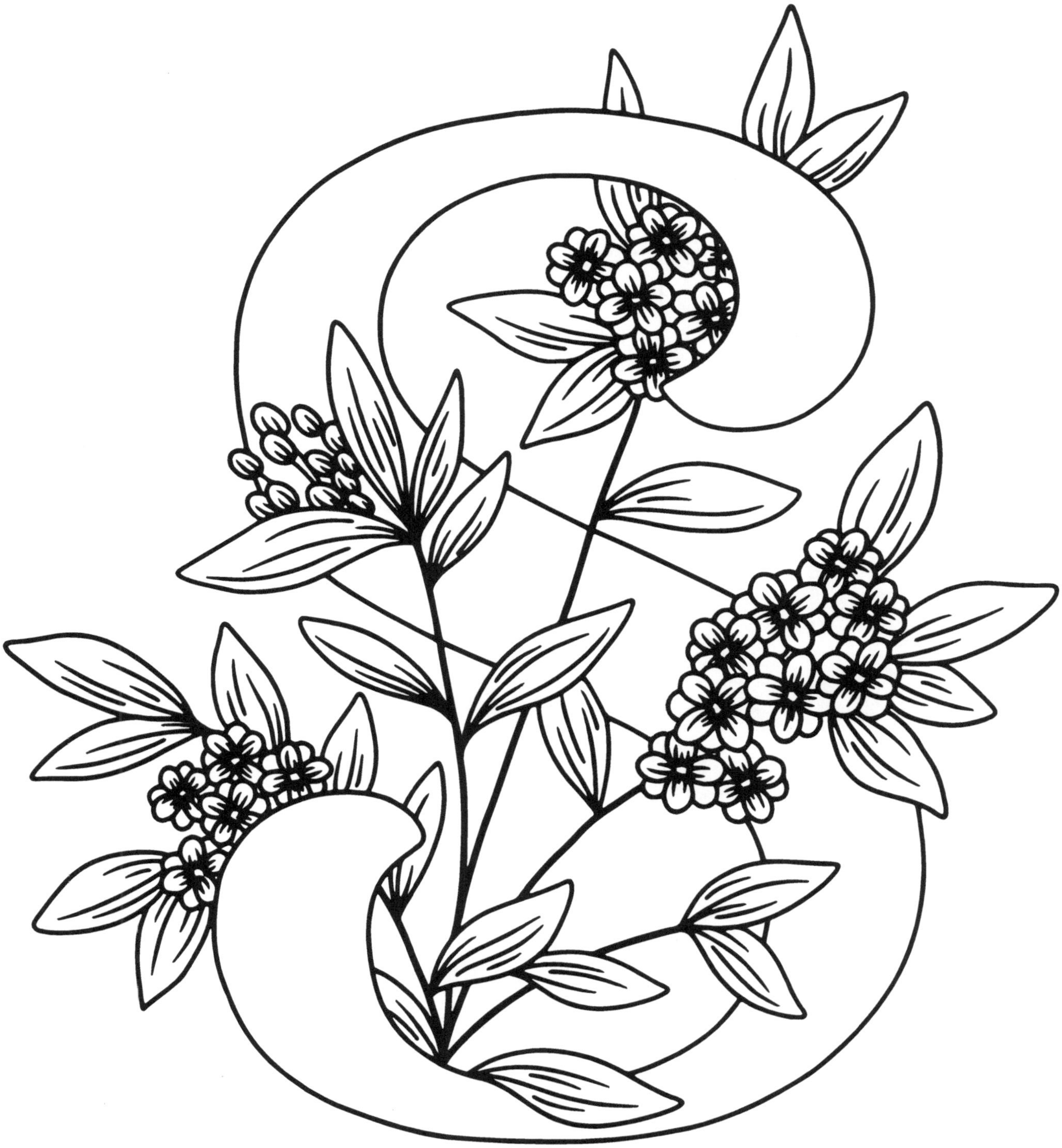

Love Letters to Hope!

Write a heartfelt letter to yourself, a loved one impacted by stomach cancer, or stomach cancer itself. Express your true feelings, thoughts, and emotions without holding back. Share messages of hope, love, or support. Let your words be a source of comfort, strength, and inspiration.

You Are Loved and Carried Through

In the midst of a stomach cancer diagnosis, it's natural to feel isolated or wonder if anyone truly understands your pain. But know this: you are deeply loved, not just by those around you, but by the love that resides within you. That inner love is a powerful force that will guide you through the darkest moments, offering comfort, peace, and strength. You are not alone in this journey. You are seen, you are heard, and you are cared for in ways that transcend words. Hold onto the love that surrounds you from family, friends, and the kindness of strangers, and the love that shines from within your own heart. You are loved more than you know.

Coloring Activity

As you navigate your stomach cancer journey, we want you to know you're loved and supported. To bring some comfort, we've included a coloring page featuring the word 'Love' and the letter L surrounded by flowers and leaves. Take a moment to pause, color, and let the peacefulness of this design wrap around you

Love

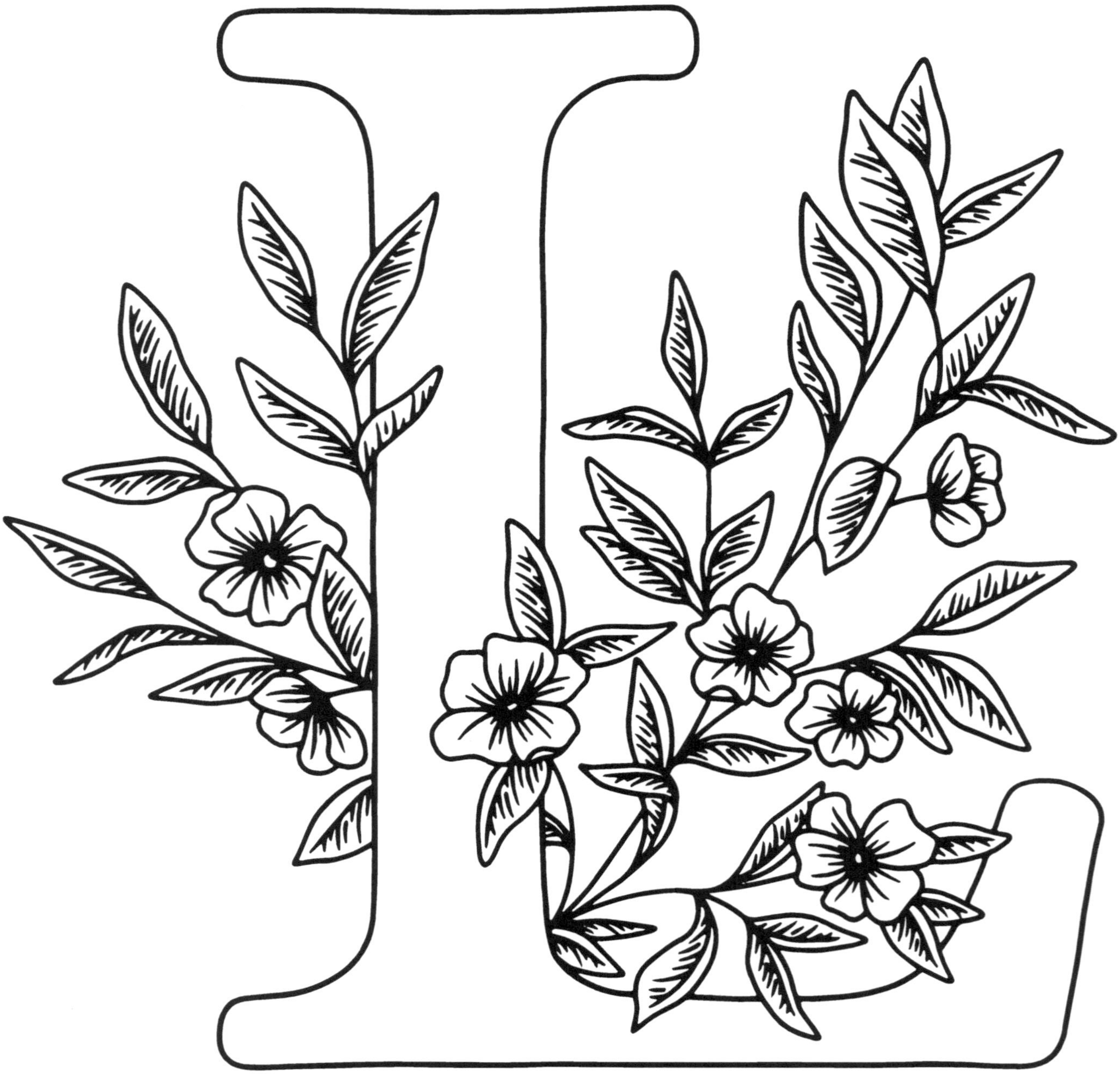

Q&A Time

QUESTION

How can I cope with the emotional impact of stomach cancer?

ANSWER

Allow yourself to feel your emotions, and don't hesitate to seek support from loved ones, support groups, or mental health professionals. Prioritize self-care activities that bring you comfort and peace.

"You never know how strong you are until being strong is the only choice you have."
~Bob Marley

STOMACH CANCER CROSSWORD PUZZLE

Read the clues below and fill in the grid.

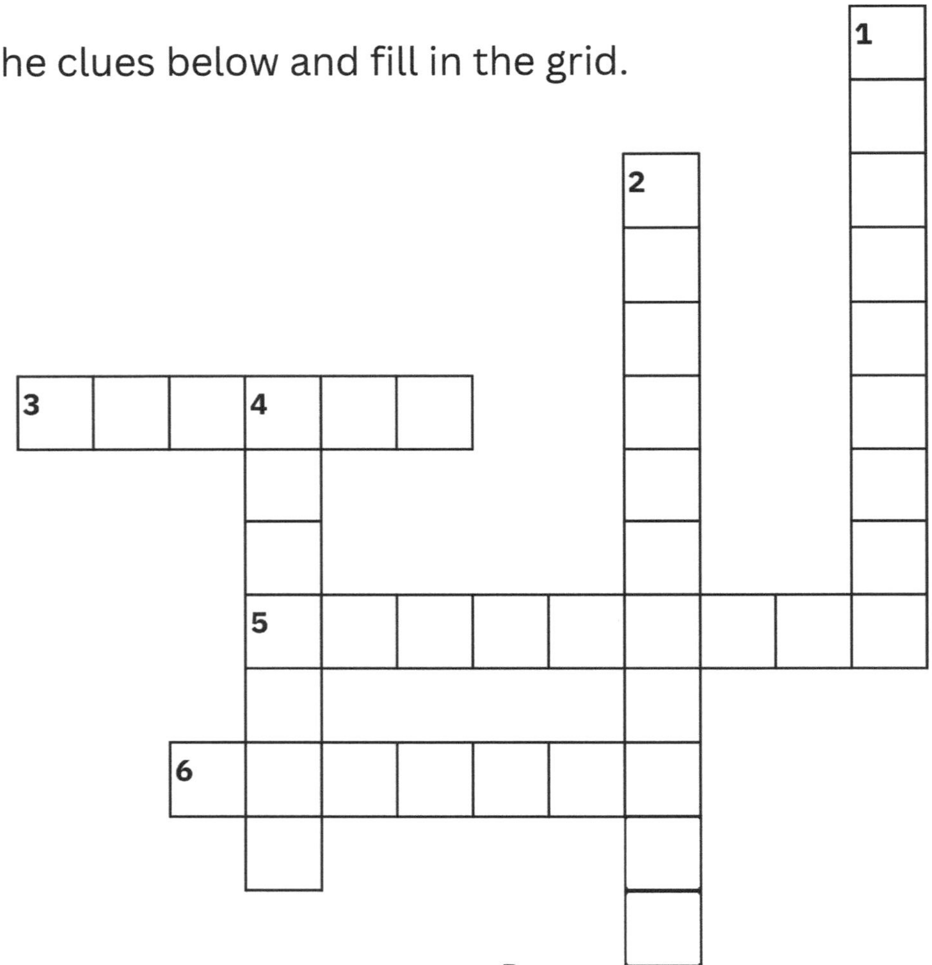

Across

3. Refers to something related to the stomach.

5. Surgery, chemotherapy, and radiation are all part of the ___ plan for stoamch cancer patents.

6. Stomach cancer patients often undergo ___ to remove tumors.

Down

1. Someone who has overcome stomach cancer is often referred to as a ___.

2. What term describes an intense and obsessive fascination with obscure or rare aspects of stomach cancer, such as unusual symptoms or potential causes?

4. When discussing a stomach cancer diagnosis with a patient, what approach is often recommended?

Nutrition and Wellness

**"DURING TREATMENT, I FOUND THAT BLAND FOODS LIKE CRACKERS,
TOAST, AND PLAIN RICE WERE EASIER
TO DIGEST. TRY KEEPING A FOOD DIARY TO TRACK WHAT WORKS AND WHAT DOESN'T FOR YOU."**

5

Nourishing Through Stomach Cancer Awareness: 5 Important Nutrients for Body Health

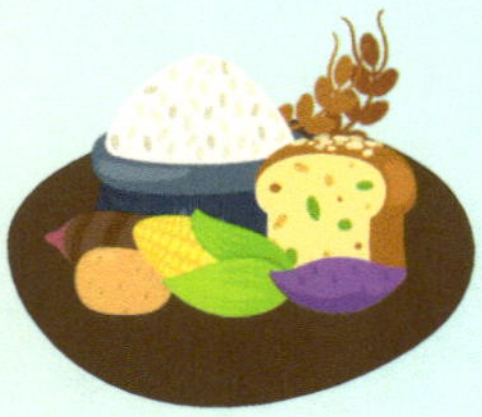

Carbohydrate

This nutrient plays a crucial role in providing energy to the body, particularly for individuals managing stomach cancer. Carbohydrates fuel the body, converting glucose into energy.

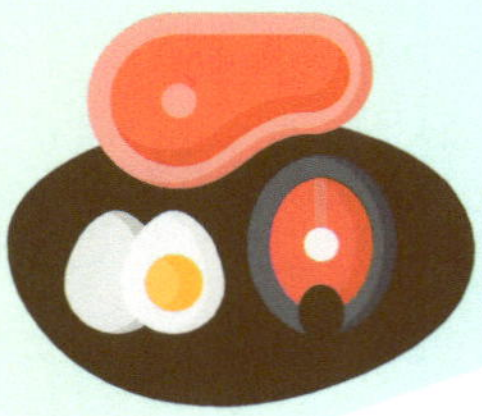

Protein

A long chain of amino acids is vital for building body blocks. Protein is very beneficial for the health of muscles, bone cells, skin, and hair during stomach cancer treatment and recovery.

Vitamins

Vitamins are crucial nutrients for various chemical processes in the body, maintaining organ function, and boosting immunity against disease during stomach cancer care.

Minerals

Minerals build strong bones and teeth, regulate metabolism, and more. Key minerals, such as calcium, iron, and zinc, are vital for overall health in the context of stomach cancer.

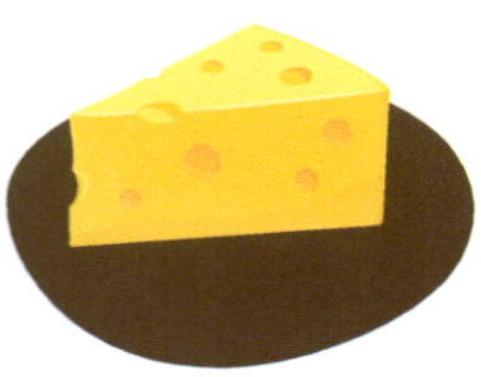

Fats

Fats maintain organ function, assist in nutrient absorption, and help with movement. Good fats can help control blood sugar and reduce heart disease risks, important considerations during stomach cancer treatment.

Food & Symptom Diary

DATE & TIME	FOOD & BEVERAGE	SYMPTOMS	NOTES

Food & Symptom Dairy

DATE & TIME	FOOD & BEVERAGE	SYMPTOMS	NOTES

Patient Empowerment Tip

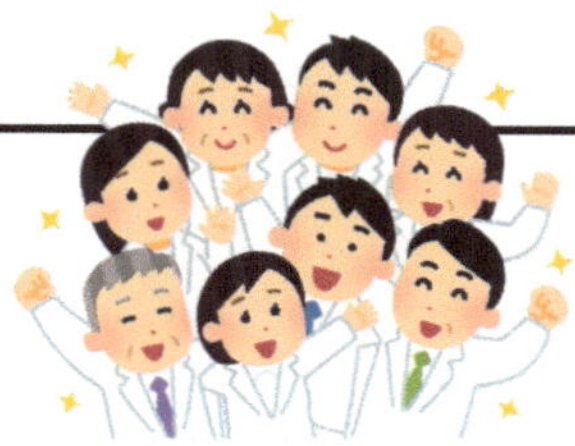

Don't be afraid to ask questions or seek a second opinion. Your healthcare team is there to support you, and it's essential to advocate for yourself throughout your journey.

RESEARCH UPDATE

New Frontiers in Stomach Cancer Treatment

Researchers are exploring new treatments for stomach cancer, including targeted therapies and immunotherapies. Stay informed about the latest developments and discuss potential options with your healthcare team.

Support System Spotlight: Shining a Light on the Heroes in Your Stomach Cancer Journey

I AM NOT ALONE

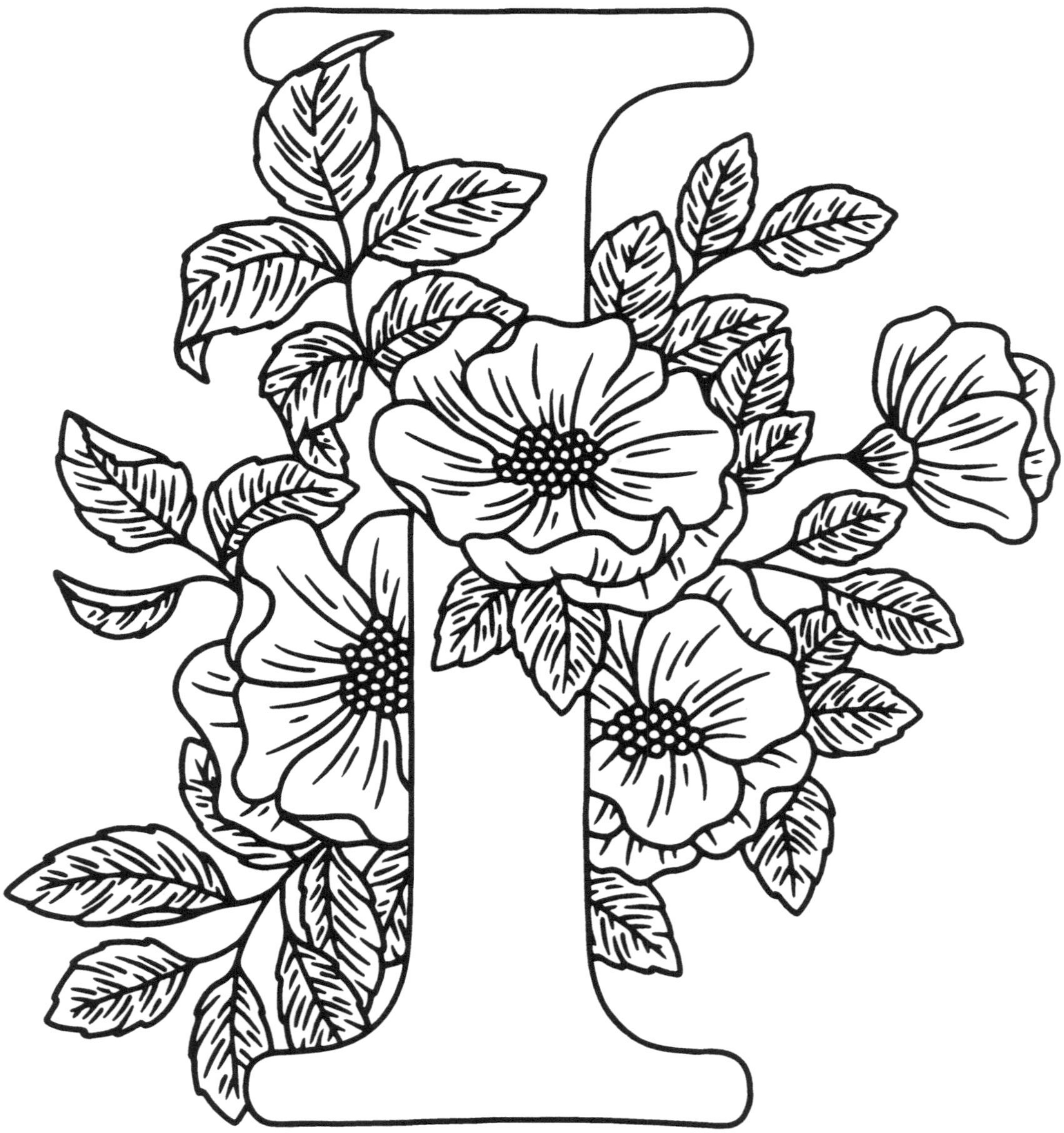

Q&A Time

QUESTION

How can I maintain hope during cancer treatment?

ANSWER

Focus on the present moment, and surround yourself with positivity. Draw inspiration from stories of survivors, and remind yourself that every day brings new opportunities for healing.

"Hope is the thing with feathers that perches in the soul and sings the tune without the words and never stops."
~Emily Dickinson

Unscramble

AFFIRMATIONS FOR THE STOMACH CANCER JOURNEY

GNTROS ______________________

PHOE ______________________

LHEA ______________________

ECRA ______________________

VLOE ______________________

TGHIF ______________________

GACREOU ______________________

HITFA ______________________

NTIESLIER ______________________

VEITSIPO ______________________

PPUSTOR ______________________

UCRE ______________________

Supporting Loved Ones with Stomach Cancer: A Guide to Making a Difference

A stomach cancer diagnosis can be a life-altering experience for both the patient and their loved ones. As a supportive partner, neighbor, friend, or family member, you can play a vital role in their journey. Here's how:

Ways to Support Your Loved One

- Emotional Support: Be present, listen to their concerns, and offer words of encouragement. Sometimes, all they need is someone to talk to.
- Practical Help: Assist with daily tasks, such as: ADLs (bathing, dressing, feeding, toileting, mobility), IADLs (meal prep, medication management, grocery shopping, household chores).
- Accompany to medical appointments: Provide emotional support and take notes during doctor visits.
- Encourage Healthy Habits: Support their nutrition and wellness goals.

Tips for Caregivers

- Take Care of Yourself: Prioritize your own physical, mental, spiritual, and emotional well-being.
- Seek Support: Reach out to friends, family, support groups, or organizations for help and guidance.
- Stay Informed: Learn about stomach cancer, its treatment options, and potential side effects.

By providing emotional support, practical help, and being informed, you can make a significant difference in your loved one's journey with stomach cancer.

Hope for Tomorrow

Take a moment to reflect on your journey with stomach cancer. Write down 3 things you hope for, whether for today, tomorrow, or the future. They can be simple (a peaceful morning, a good conversation with a loved one) or big (successful treatment, a milestone celebration).

Hope

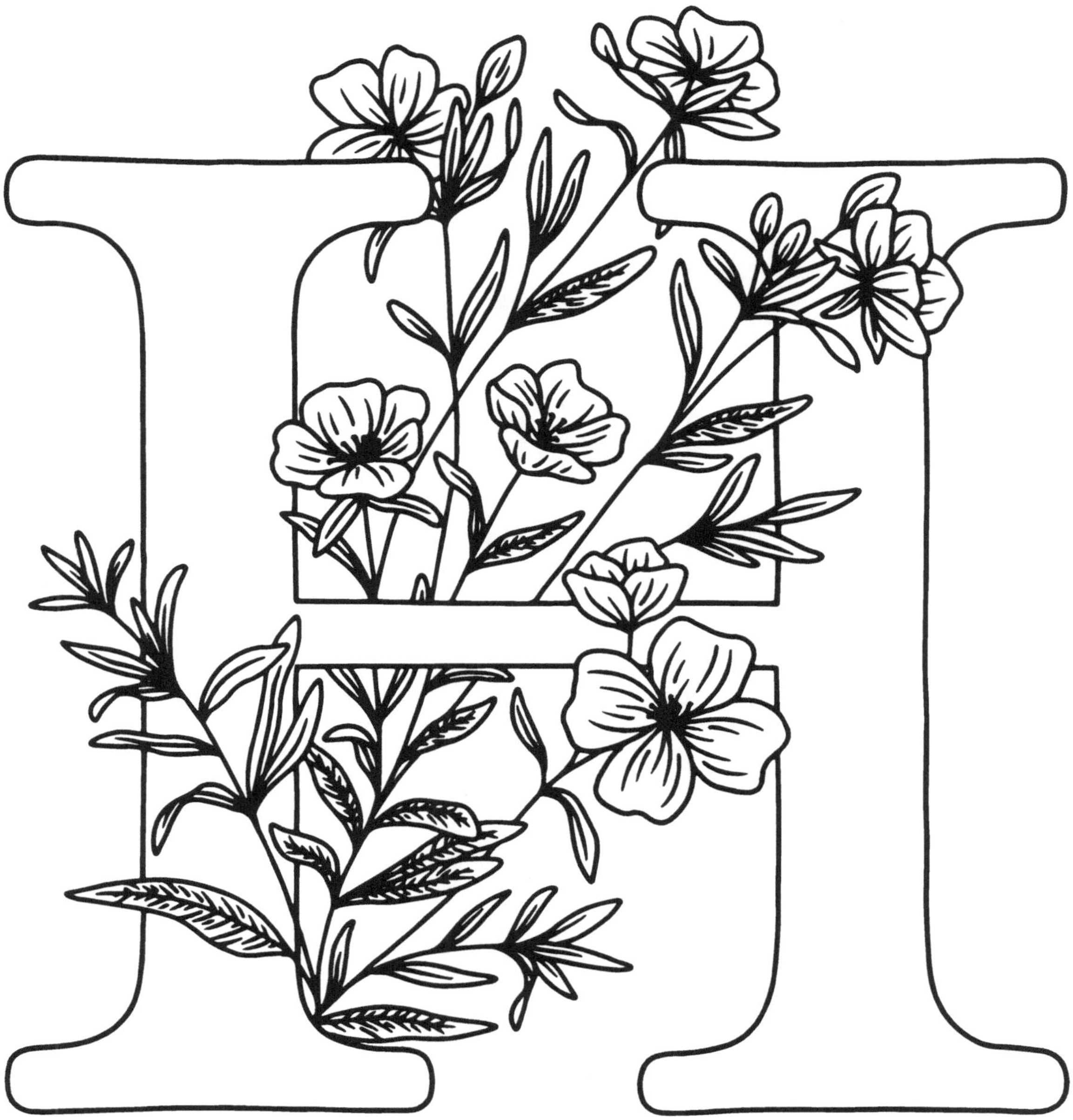

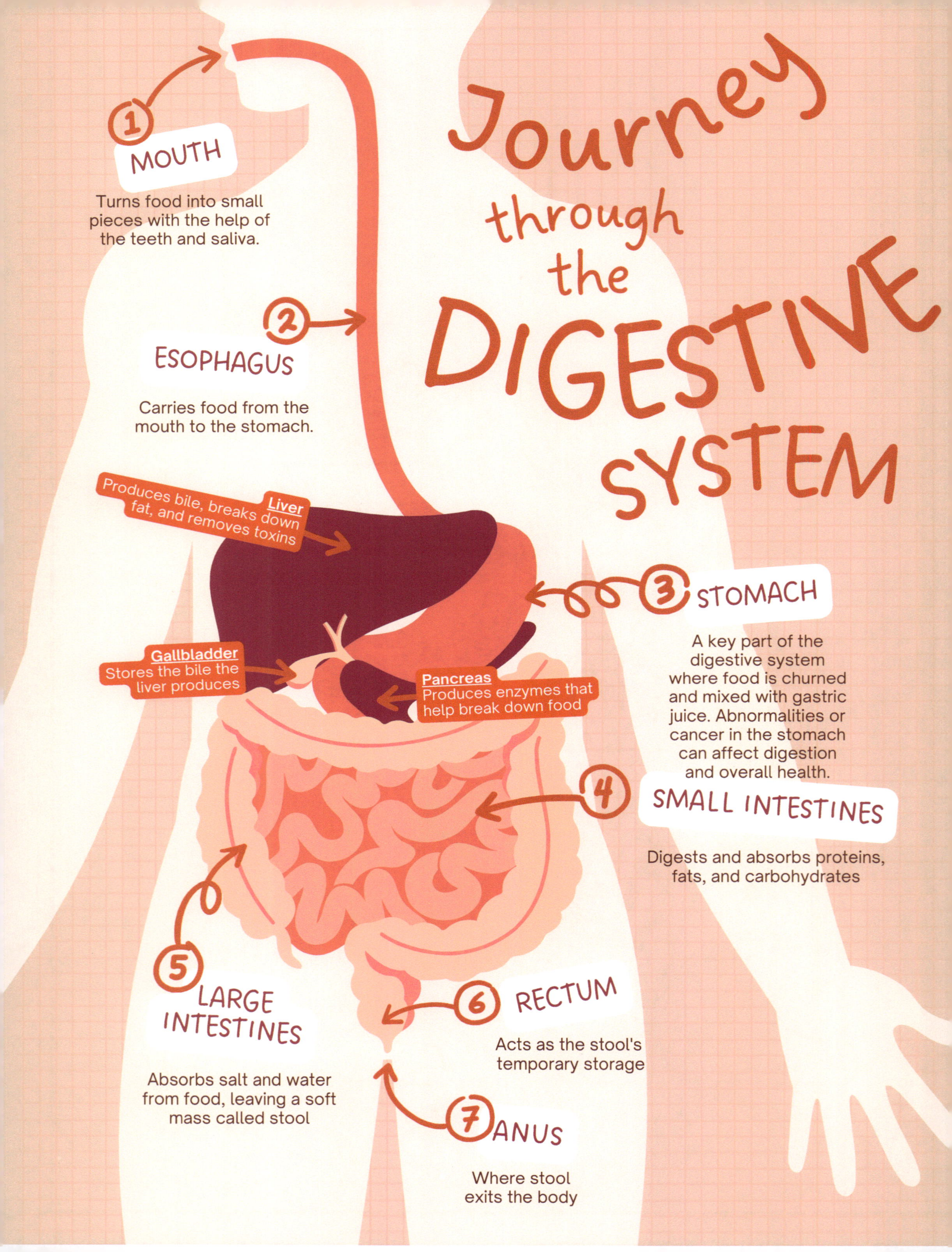
Journey through the DIGESTIVE SYSTEM
1
MOUTH
Turns food into small pieces with the help of the teeth and saliva.
2
ESOPHAGUS
Carries food from the mouth to the stomach.
Liver
Produces bile, breaks down fat, and removes toxins
3
STOMACH
A key part of the digestive system where food is churned and mixed with gastric juice. Abnormalities or cancer in the stomach can affect digestion and overall health.
Gallbladder
Stores the bile the liver produces
Pancreas
Produces enzymes that help break down food
4
SMALL INTESTINES
Digests and absorbs proteins, fats, and carbohydrates
5
LARGE INTESTINES
Absorbs salt and water from food, leaving a soft mass called stool
6
RECTUM
Acts as the stool's temporary storage
7
ANUS
Where stool exits the body

Connecting the Digestive System to Stomach Cancer

Label the digestive system diagram, and explain each structure's function. Discuss how stomach cancer affects the stomach, other parts of the digestive system, and overall health.

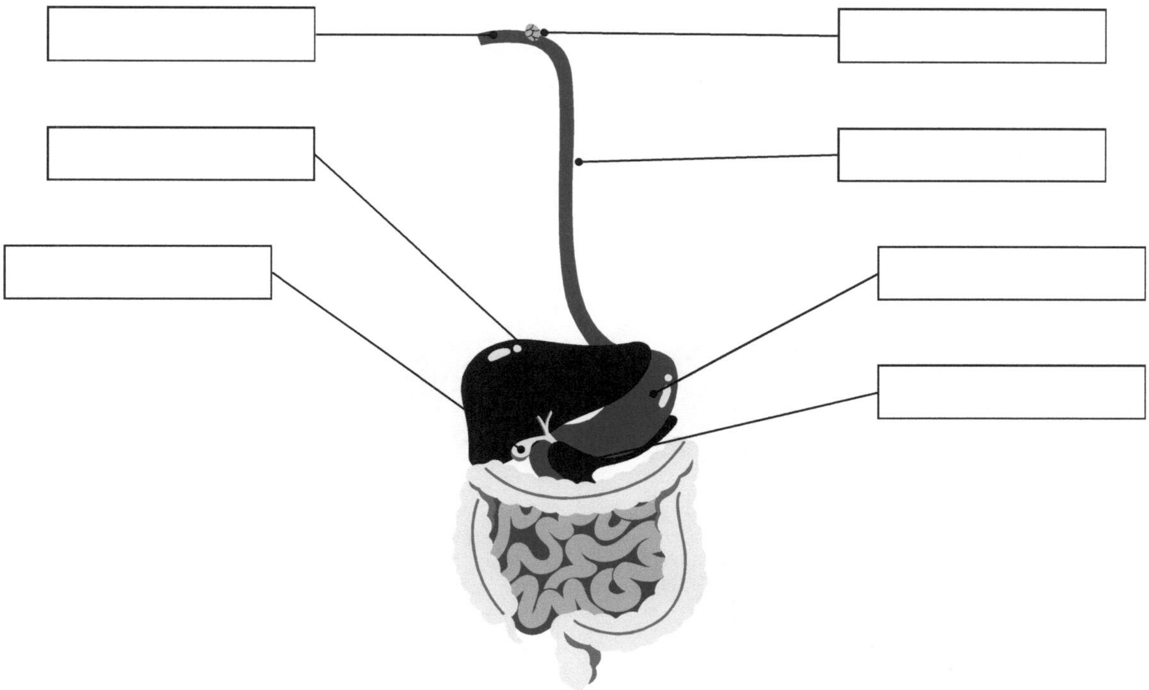

Structure	Function
mouth	
salivary glades	
esophagus	
liver	
stomach	
gallbladder	
pancreas	

Quick Tip

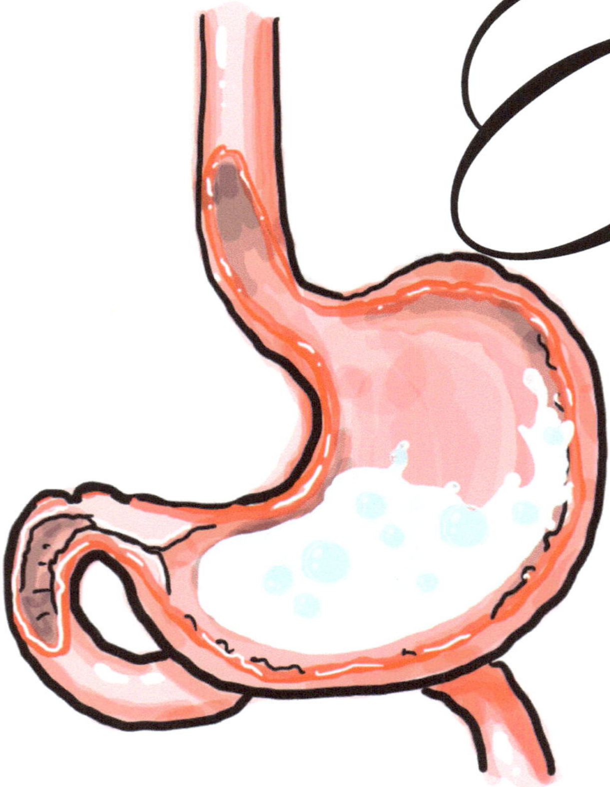

DID YOU KNOW THAT STOMACH CANCER IS MORE COMMON IN MEN THAN IN WOMEN?

ACCORDING TO THE AMERICAN CANCER SOCIETY, MEN ARE ABOUT 1.7 TIMES MORE LIKELY TO DEVELOP STOMACH CANCER THAN WOMEN.

APA REFERENCE:

AMERICAN CANCER SOCIETY. (2025). _*KEY STATISTICS ABOUT STOMACH CANCER*. RETRIEVED FROM HTTPS://WWW.CANCER.ORG/CANCER/STOMACH-CANCER/ABOUT/KEY-STATISTICS.HTML

SURVIVOR TIPS

During my treatment, I found that staying hydrated and eating small, frequent meals helped manage my symptoms.

~Sarah

Stomach Cancer Survivor

As a caregiver, it’s essential to take breaks and prioritize your own self-care. Managing stress through activities such as reading, walking, or practicing yoga can help you support your loved one more effectively.

Don't overlook your own needs.

The most successful awareness campaigns for stomach cancer aren’t about being loud. It’s about being the message, such as emphasizing the importance of early detection, and repeating it often to build understanding and support.

Cancer Wish List

Write down your wishes, hopes, or prayers.

STOMACH CANCER SELF-CARE COMPASS

EVEN ON BAD DAYS

Soak Away Treatment Fatigue	Calming Tunes for Chemo Days	Journal My Journey Through Chemo
Breathe Fresh Air After Treatment	Find Strength in Gentle Stretches	Warmth in a Cup During Recovery
Treat yourself to a favorite snack	Movie Night for Cancer Fatigue	Lean on Loved Ones During Surgery Recovery

Q&A Time

QUESTION

How can I overcome my fear of cancer recurrence?

ANSWER

Remember that navigating cancer is a journey with ups and downs. Focus on what you can learn from your experience and how you've grown through treatment and recovery rather than just the outcome.

"Courage doesn't always roar. Sometimes courage is the quiet voice at the end of the day saying, "I will try again tomorrow."
-Mary Anne Radmacher

Sarah wants to write about her journey with stomach cancer; she's using her story to process emotions and inspire others.

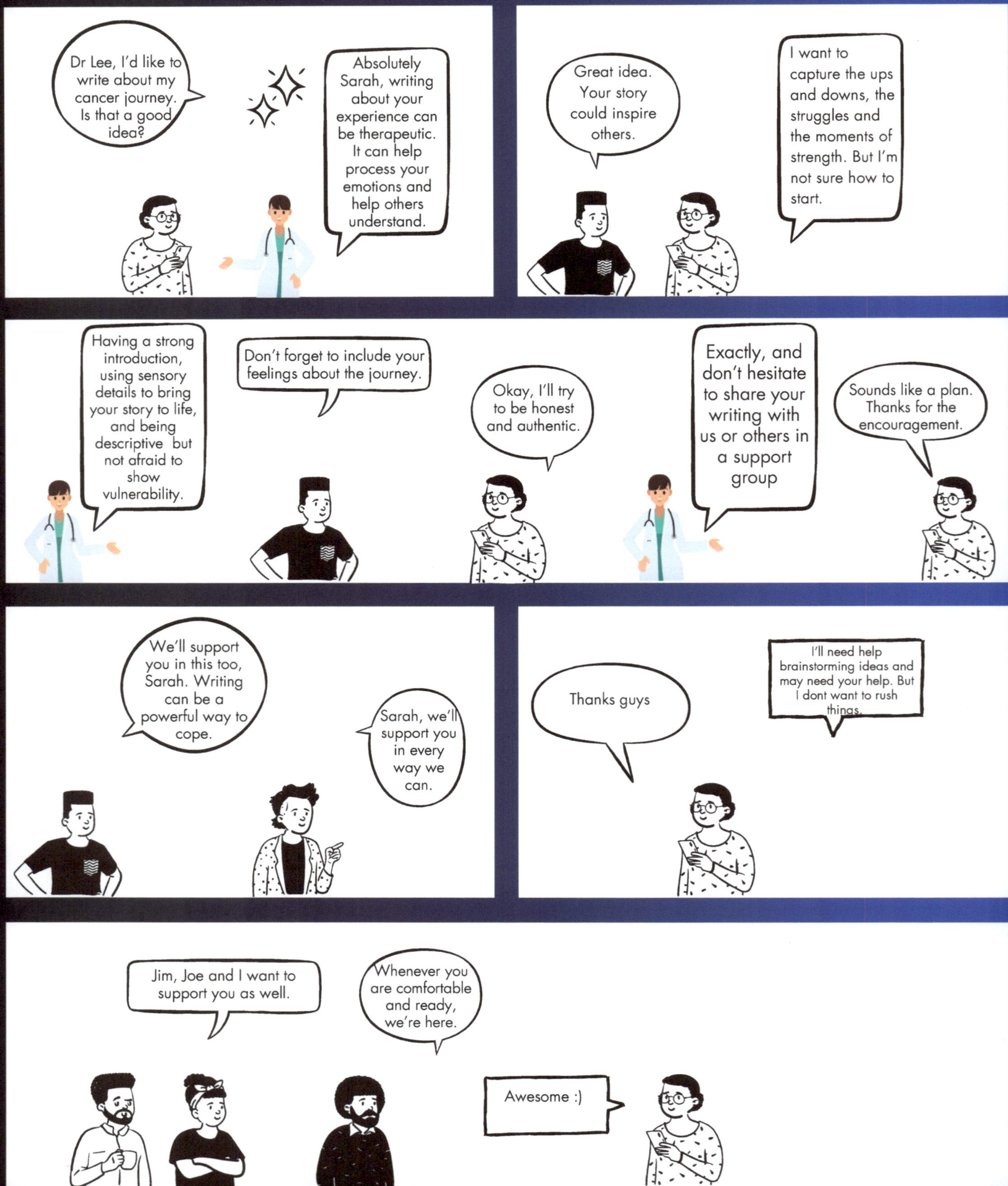

Dr Lee, I'd like to write about my cancer journey. Is that a good idea?
Absolutely Sarah, writing about your experience can be therapeutic. It can help process your emotions and help others understand.
Great idea. Your story could inspire others.
I want to capture the ups and downs, the struggles and the moments of strength. But I'm not sure how to start.
Having a strong introduction, using sensory details to bring your story to life, and being descriptive but not afraid to show vulnerability.
Don't forget to include your feelings about the journey.
Okay, I'll try to be honest and authentic.
Exactly, and don't hesitate to share your writing with us or others in a support group
Sounds like a plan. Thanks for the encouragement.
We'll support you in this too, Sarah. Writing can be a powerful way to cope.
Sarah, we'll support you in every way we can.
Thanks guys
I'll need help brainstorming ideas and may need your help. But I dont want to rush things.
Jim, Joe and I want to support you as well.
Whenever you are comfortable and ready, we're here.
Awesome :)

Let's Talk:

Fostering Supportive Dialogues for Stomach Cancer Warriors at Work

Creating a supportive work envoirnment for individuals with stomach cancer.

How are you really doing with your treatment?

Is there anything I can do to support you?

What can we do to help you feel more comfortable?

How can we accommodate your needs at work?

What do you need from us to make things easier while you're going through treatment?

Start the conversation. Support each other. Together, we build a healthier workplace. Let's work together to create a culture of empathy, understanding, and support.

Love Letters

LOVE LETTERS CAN PROVIDE EMOTIONAL SUPPORT AND COMFORT. OFFERING A PERSONAL AND RELATABLE PERSPECTIVE ON THE STOMACH CANCER EXPERIENCE. LOVE LETTERS INSPIRE HOPE, RESILIENCE, AND COURAGE. LOVE LETTERS EXPRESS GRATITUDE AND APPRECIATION FOR CAREGIVERS, FAMILY, AND FRIENDS. THEY CREATE A SENSE OF CONNECTION.

DEAR SELF

I'm so proud of you for fighting through the darkest days. Your strength and resilience inspire me every day. Remember to be gentle with yourself and celebrate every small victory.

WITH LOVE AND ADMIRATION

DEAR FAMILY AND FRIENDS

Thank you for being my rock during this journey. Your love, support, and encouragement mean the world to me. I'm grateful for every hug, every listening ear, and every helping hand.

WITH LOVE AND APPRECIATION

DEAR CAREGIVERS

Your compassion, kindess, and expertise
have been a ray of light for me.
Thank you for holding my hand through
the toughest moments and for helping
me navigate this journey. I apologize if I
have been rude to you or out of line.
Please forgive me

WITH GRATITUDE AND RESPECT.

DEAR FELLOW WARRIORS

You are not alone in this fight. Hold on to hope, even when the road ahead seems uncertain. Your strength inspires others, and your story matters.

WITH LOVE AND SOLIDARITY

STOMACH CANCER GLOSSARY: KEY MEDICAL TERMS DEFINED

Use this glossary as a resource to enhance your understanding of stomach cancer and its treatment options.

	Medical Term	Medical Meaning
C	Chemotherapy	Treatment that uses drugs to stop the growth of cells.
P	Port	An impacted device through which blood can be taken and medication can be given.
R	Radiation	Treatment that uses high-energy rays to kill cells and/or shrink tumors.
T	Tumor	An abnormal mass of tissue that comes from the overgrowth of cells.
G	Gastric	Relating to the stomach.

	Medical Term	Medical Meaning
B	Biopsy	A procedure where a sample of tissue is removed from the stomach and examined under a microscope to check for cancer cells.
E	Endoscopy	A procedure that uses a flexible tube with a camera and light to visually examine the inside of the stomach and digestive tract.
M	Metastasis	The spread of cancer cells from the stomach to other parts of the body.
G	Gastrectomy	Surgical removal of part or all of the stomach
A	Adenocarcinoma	Most common type of stomach cancer

Understanding medical terms can empower patients to make informed decisions about their treatment plan. It improves communication with your healthcare providers, helps navigate medical reports, and can reduce anxiety. By being informed, patients can take an active role in their care and make decisions that are best suited to them.

Thank You

A Message of Appreciation & Hope

Dear Friends and Supporters,

I want to express my heartfelt gratitude to each of you for taking the time to engage with this booklet, and for being part of the effort
to bring awareness, knowledge, and hope to those affected by stomach cancer.
Every small step we take together helps to spread understanding, encourage support,
and uplift those who need it most.

As a loved one, I've seen firsthand the impact that stomach cancer can have on
individuals and families. But I've also seen the power of hope, resilience,
and community in the face of adversity. By sharing this booklet with others,
we can spark conversations, provide comfort, and remind those
affected that they are not alone.

I invite you to continue exploring resources that can inspire reflection,
healing and growth.

With Gratitude, Hope,
and Love ♡

Delatria Tam

IN LOVING MEMORY

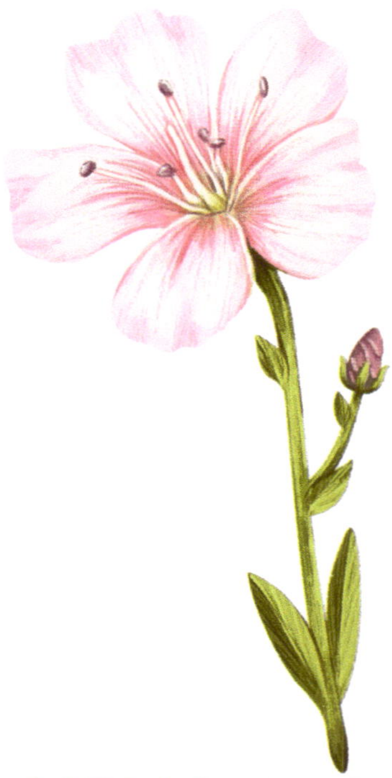

IN LOVING MEMORY OF MY LOVED ONE, WHO PASSED AWAY DUE TO STOMACH CANCER. YOUR LOVE, BRAVERY, STRENGTH, AND RESILIENCE WILL NEVER BE FORGOTTEN.

www.ingramcontent.com/pod-product-compliance
Lightning Source LLC
LaVergne TN
LVHW070955210926
848482LV00002B/221

* 9 7 9 8 3 4 9 5 6 7 5 0 6 *